EATING DISORDER RECOVERY

PARENT HANDBOOK

TOUGH
COOKIE

First Printing: February 2016

ISBN: 978-1-326-55051-6

Tough Cookie Publishing

Email: info@toughcookieblog.co.uk

www.toughcookieblog.co.uk

Ordering Information:

Special discounts are available on quantity purchases by corporations, associations, educators, and others. For details, please contact the publisher at the above listed address.

U.S. trade bookstores and wholesalers: Please contact Tough Cookie Publishing at the above listed address.

Special thanks to Alison and John Walters for your input in this book, and for your unconditional love and support as always.

Contents

1. About Me

I founded Tough Cookie because I recovered from Anorexia myself at the age of fourteen, and after getting through it alone, I still see many struggling with little or no support. With so many negative influences online and in the media I wanted to bring something positive and accessible to the table. My experience is specifically with Anorexia and more recently anxiety and body dysmorphic disorder, but I hope to use the things I've learnt (and am still learning!) to help people with all kinds of eating disorders.

I also hear a lot of people saying that they do well in hospital on specialist units and feel better in that environment, but struggle or relapse once they are home with little or no support. Tough Cookie is about changing that – through helping people to help themselves, and teaching others how to support them in doing so.

Following my illness I wanted to help others but also campaign for better awareness and the prevention of eating disorders through positive mental wellbeing, better body image and early intervention. I regularly speak to schools, professional groups and young people about self-esteem, nutrition and eating disorders and I've written several other books to help people who are going through the same experiences I did to offer my personal insight and the things I have discovered which have helped me to live my life to the full.

2. About this book

I believe that an important part of helping others with eating disorders is reaching their parents and families. My parents were an instrumental element of my recovery from Anorexia – and I absolutely know that without them, I might not be here today. It's so hard for the people left locked on the outside of an eating disorder, because the person they love is disappearing physically and mentally and they often feel powerless to do anything about it.

As well as providing support for people going through eating disorders, I also wanted to recognise and support parents in their incredibly important and crucial role. That's why I decided to write a separate handbook specifically for parents, which uses my own experience and shares insights from my parents to help you to understand the illness better, to know what to do, what to say and to show you that you're not alone in what you are going through.

I felt this book was essential because more often than not, it's the young person's family who are on the front line fighting for their loved one as they are unable at first to fight for themselves. With few resources to help people with eating disorders and a lack of urgency and understanding, many cases worsen as they are left to exacerbate – with parents and family members standing by helplessly watching the person they love suffer. I know first-hand from speaking to my own parents that it is so frustrating and desperately worrying when access to help and support seems to be continually out of reach. When this is combined with unwillingness to access support from the person in question due to the nature of the illness, it can be incredibly difficult for family and friends to know what is best to do and how to help them.

This book should hopefully answer some of the questions you have about your child's condition and how you can help them and support them through this whilst taking care of yourself. I've included personal insights from my own experience which I share with professionals and parents alike, with specific chapters including details of my own recovery and insights into what it's like to suffer with and overcome an eating disorder. I also worked closely with my parents on this book and they contribute throughout to ensure that it is as comprehensive and authentic as possible – as whilst I appreciate what an eating disorder is like for your child, I can't fully understand how it must have felt from my parents' perspective.

This is why their input is invaluable, as whilst I can share my perspective now and insights from the experience at the time, they went through what you are going through personally and can offer their own advice and support. You'll find quotes from them throughout the book.

At the end of the book you'll also find a list of charities and organisations which you may find useful, but for further reading or to get in touch please visit my website below.

www.toughcookieblog.co.uk

3. What is an eating disorder?

As eating disorders are more prevalent in the press now, you might already feel you have a good understanding of what the definition of an eating disorder is. In this book I go over the general information which you may know already, but I also offer my own personal insight from the perspective of someone who has been there and actually experienced an eating disorder first hand. I had Anorexia, so my personal experience is limited to that alone, but this book covers both Anorexia and Bulimia specifically.

What is an eating disorder?

An eating disorder is defined as a psychological illness causing the sufferer to have abnormal eating habits or exhibit unusual behaviour regarding food and eating. The term actually covers a wide range of mental illnesses which cause abnormal activity around food, including Anorexia, Bulimia and binge eating disorders. This book covers Anorexia and Bulimia, which are described below:

Anorexia

A person with Anorexia aims to keep their weight as low as possible – even when their weight and BMI are dangerously low and seriously affect their mental and physical health. This involves self-starvation, limiting general food intake, refusing to eat certain foods and sometimes refusing to drink. People with Anorexia will often also exercise excessively to 'burn off' food, even when they are very weak. The effects of Anorexia long-term can be devastating, with brittle bones, infertility, severe hair loss and digestive damage sometimes caused when someone is underweight for a prolonged length of time.

Bulimia

A person with Bulimia may also aim to be a low weight or control their weight, but rather than starvation they go through periods of binge eating which is followed by 'purging'. Purging involves the person deliberately making themselves sick or using laxatives to dispose of the food eaten quickly before it has had chance to be fully absorbed by the body. Whilst a person with Anorexia may hide or limit food, people with Bulimia may appear to eat normally or even excessively, but still lose weight as a consequence of purging everything they eat. Bulimia can also have devastating consequences both in the short and long term for sufferers – including dental complications, significant digestive problems, brittle bones, infertility and hair loss amongst the medical issues caused following the illness.

Anorexia and Bulimia can be present together or can feature elements of one another – for example, a person with Bulimia may also exercise excessively, and a person with Anorexia may sometimes purge to get rid of food they have been forced to eat. Predominantly eating disorders affect women, but men can and do also develop eating disorders.

Both Anorexia and Bulimia are very serious conditions and often arise out of a need for control. They can be caused by the sufferer feeling 'fat' and wishing to be slim or to lose weight, but that's not always the case. Anorexia used to be known as 'the slimmer's disease' – and it's this and largely false media that has led people to believe the misconception that eating disorders are all about food and body image, when in fact there are many other causes and triggers behind them. There is more on this in **Chapter 5**.

My experience with Anorexia

I often talk candidly about my experience with Anorexia in my books and talks, as I believe that the only way to help others to understand and overcome the illness is to be open and honest about every part of the illness, and everything I went through during and after recovery.

I developed Anorexia because I was bullied at school predominantly for being fat (but also over a number of other things) all day, every day. I was already struggling with severe OCD, which ended up helping me get picked on even more. I eventually became tired of the hurt and emotional pain I suffered constantly and I hated myself – I just desperately wanted to fit in and I believed that there must be something wrong with me for me to be treated this way by everybody at school with no respite.

I started to become obsessed with reading celebrity magazines and newspapers – in particular I liked to read the 'diet advice' and learn about celebrity weights and eating habits. One day I saw an article about Anorexia with 'before and after' pictures. It seemed like a simple yet perfect solution to me - if I could lose a lot of weight, all I would need to do is put a little back on, so I wouldn't be the person I was before (who I believed was wrong in every way possible, disliked by everybody and 'fat'), but I would instead be healthy and slim and beautiful and smiling in a magazine talking about my journey and being praised by others. This is exactly how it looked to me – but of course it wasn't like that at all, and for me to see it that way, I must already have been poorly. I had an ignorance and lack of understanding of the illness, as so many people do. I didn't realise that it wasn't something I could control – and in fact it took me years to realise that it was in fact controlling me, and not the other way around.

When you have an eating disorder, you become so obsessed with food that it consumes you; it's all you think about. You have no time for anything, or anyone, else. You become a shell of a person, you become angry and irritable. As you eat less, your brain (as well as other major organs) stops functioning properly. That means it becomes harder to think clearly, resulting in you becoming more and more irrational. Logic, rationality and ability to reason disappear.

I have always described Anorexia (I can't speak for Bulimia, however I imagine it is very similar) as a demon inside my head. I was still there; my personality, my humility, everything I loved in life. Yet slowly I had been replaced; my brain had been taken over by another entity whose sole focus was to destroy me. To kill me, ultimately. This demon told me I was better off dead. It convinced me that I was disliked because I was fat and ugly and anything other than my current state (morbidly underweight) constituted that (fat and ugly); therefore I could either be unlovable or die. It had to be one of the two – there appeared to be nothing in between. I was miserable and incredibly poorly physically, but I was controlled fearfully by my illness.

Relatives and friends told me to 'just eat'. And whilst I wanted to, this parasite inside my head strongly advised me not to and I had no way of escaping the fear it had instilled in me of leading a normal life.

Food became an enemy, and along with it so did everybody around me who tried to help. But because the demon got angry with my family and friends, they got angry back. They felt helpless and frustrated and a lot of professional people who were supposed to be helping me directed cruel words at me or pointed the finger at my family, who were desperately trying to get me back.

My personality had completely disappeared by the time I was at my lowest weight – I was just drifting around, a shell of who I used to be, unable to talk or smile or think properly. The only thing occupying my mind was how I was going to avoid the next time someone tried to get me to eat or drink something. I started to wonder whether the air I breathed contained calories. Very much wishing I could just die - knowing I was nearly there. Inside, the 'real me' was frightened and guilty.

It took a long while for me to realise that I was worth a shot, and to decide I wanted to live a proper life. It was a journey of ups and downs – some days I felt it deserved to live, other days I simply wanted to die. I believe it was constant encouragement from people around me, little things that they did and said which slowly but surely made a huge difference in my mind. I started to want things that I just couldn't have if I weighed just a few stone and lived in a hospital. It was the most difficult thing I ever did but I look back now with immense gratitude for having been able to come through it, not without lingering scars and difficulties, but without relapse and in a position to be able to help others.

How I describe an eating disorder

As I mention above, I describe Anorexia specifically (as this is what I have personal experience of) as a parasitic demon because for me it was almost like being trapped inside my own brain with something which wanted me to die and convinced me that I was better off if I followed its instructions without exception.

I realised when I was doing final edits on my other book, Tough Cookie, that every time I talked about Anorexia I had personalised and personified it, and kept referring to it as another human being. I think this is because that's almost how it was for me – like having another person in control of me inside my own head – a person who I couldn't ignore because they seemed to make a lot of sense.

Anorexia can be schizophrenic in that sense – a loud, vicious voice in your head which has a personality all of its own – a personality which terrifyingly comes out in the words you speak and the things you do. My mum likened it to me being possessed when I said certain things which were completely out of character or screamed at her calling her a bitch because she was trying to help me by making me food. I don't think many people see this side of Anorexia – or talk about it – which is why I think it's important to share it in this book. I talk more about differentiating between your child and the eating disorder inside them later on in **Chapter 7.**

Common Misconceptions

'An eating disorder is a choice'

A common misconception about eating disorders is that the person involved has a choice and has wilfully made a decision not to eat. It's simple – it's solely about food and the person's apparent choice not to eat it. When I was poorly it didn't occur to many people that Anorexia wasn't a choice – just as cancer and MS aren't choices. It is a very difficult thing for people to get their heads around – and I was often attacked by family members, medical staff, even strangers - which is why I do what I do with a goal of using my own experience to explain Anorexia to others.

Eating disorders are not self-inflicted; it is not a choice to have an eating disorder. Because it masquerades as the individual in question, it's easy to come to that conclusion. The words come out of their mouth; the actions are made by them. But what I and others who have had or currently have an eating disorder know is that it's not really you, and it's very hard for others (and sometimes for you yourself) to differentiate between what's you and what's the eating.

Nobody should **ever** make anyone feel guilty for having had an eating disorder, just as it would be unthinkable to accuse somebody with cancer or MS or Parkinson's of 'ruining someone's life' or being 'selfish'.

'Eating disorders are self-indulgent'

When we believe that sufferers have a choice, that's when we conclude that they are clearly doing what they are doing for some selfish reason.

How *selfish* that person must be to put their loved ones through so much pain – to take up valuable healthcare resources, when they could just eat.

Far from a cry for attention, eating disorders are dangerous, complex and much more serious than a refusal to eat.

'Eating disorders can't be overcome'

This is **untrue** and I am living proof of that – along with lots of others who have recovered and continue to recover fully without relapse. However the numbers of people achieving this are way too low.

I believe that when we focus on conventional methods and discount everything else, we close the door to recovery for so many people. This combined with a lack of understanding is what makes Anorexia so deadly. But if we spread understanding and encourage recovery through any method possible, we can make a difference.

In Tough Cookie, I talk about conventional therapy, but I also stress that if this 'hasn't worked' (for whatever reason – maybe the therapist or timing wasn't quite right, or the therapy wasn't appropriate) – there are alternatives and they *can* still get better.

I include alternative tools and ways of thinking for people struggling with eating disorders in Tough Cookie for this reason – some of which I'll go into more detail about (along with how you can help) in **Chapter 8**.

'Eating disorders are a product of weakness'

Weak people don't get eating disorders. You have to be very strong in fact, I believe, to carry something like this on your shoulders. Invariably sufferers go on and on and on – even those who sadly eventually pass – for months, years in an emaciated state. Some go to work, go about their daily lives, hiding what's going on for unimaginable periods of time. These are not the actions of weak people. These are the actions of people who are poorly beyond belief, consumed by an eating disorder, who desperately want to be right in some way but feel all wrong.

'Eating disorders are all about food'

People tend to think that an eating disorder is all about food – the person just 'won't' or 'can't' eat and they need to be encouraged to eat again. This is probably because it heavily involves food and also involves the person losing weight. But an eating disorder is not just about food – it's so much more than that. It's not about being faddy, awkward, stubborn or being on an 'extreme diet'.

Food is the product – unusual habits around food are the resulting behaviour, so it's easy to assume that food is the root. But actually the root can be a number of things. Low self-esteem, negative beliefs, OCD, anxiety and depression can be behind an eating disorder. To give an example, the root of my eating disorder was pretty much all of the above plus natural perfectionism. Because I was bullied for being fat and ugly day in day out at such a young age, I believed that – so I also believed I was a bad person, not worthy of other people's affection or a life like anyone else's. When I went on a diet I did so to lose weight to be liked, but I soon became disillusioned with my slow progress and when I saw eating disorders glamourised in the press I thought that restricting my food intake must be the way forward – because then I could be like these popular celebrities. I soon became 'addicted' to losing weight and a few favourable comments from the bullies at school spurred me along. So although the result was Anorexia, the root cause was that I was very unhappy inside – I hated myself.

Once you realise that an eating disorder is not a choice, everything I've discussed above should seem obvious. Please never make the assumption that someone is weak, selfish, inconsiderate or stupid because they have an eating disorder – and if you hear people saying otherwise, correct them using the things you will learn reading this book.

4. How do I know if my child has an eating disorder?

The signs of an eating disorder are often quite subtle, but can develop rapidly and quickly increase in intensity over a short period of time. Watch out for the signs such as secretive behaviour, a lack of desire to eat around others, not wanting to go out to dinner or be in a situation where they cannot control their food, and of course the obvious symptoms such as getting thinner and excessive exercise. Eventually these symptoms are so intense that it is impossible to misconstrue them for anything other than an eating disorder.

Because eating disorders are secretive by nature, it can be incredibly difficult to know for sure whether there is something wrong. It's highly unlikely that your child will tell you they are starving themselves, over-exercising, hiding food or making themselves sick.

You may already know for sure that your child has an eating disorder or have a definitive diagnosis, but for those who are unsure, this chapter should be helpful. It's very important to ensure that a change in behaviour or physical weight loss really is an eating disorder before you approach your child. The signs however do tend to be quite noticeable once you know what to look out for, and you can find some of these on the following page.

Symptoms of Anorexia

Symptoms of Anorexia include:

- Eating very little, avoiding fatty, sugary or high-carb foods, obsessively controlling food intake
- Missing meals and avoiding meal times
- Not allowing others to prepare food – or needing to know what is contained within meals cooked by others
- Anxiety and stress over eating out or situations in which they have little control over what they eat
- Lying about having eaten or hiding food
- Obsessively counting calories in food and an obsessive attitude around food and eating, including the scrutiny of others' eating habits
- Irritability – especially when questioned about food or their behaviour
- Repeatedly weighing or checking in the mirror – with unrealistic expectation and perspective of their body size and image
- Looking physically thinner
- Weakness, dizziness, hair loss and dry skin - symptoms associated with the physical side effects of starvation
- Isolation – losing interest in doing the things they used to love or seeing other people

Anorexia can be accompanied by other mental illnesses, such as OCD, anxiety, depression, self-harm and low self-esteem as well as alcohol and drug abuse.

Symptoms of Bulimia

Symptoms of Bulimia include:

- Obsessive behaviour around food and eating
- Unrealistic, distorted sense of body size and shape
- Isolation – losing interest in doing the things they love to do and seeing other people
- Anxiety over mealtimes
- Buying laxatives
- Rushing to the toilet or disappearing after each mealtime

As with Anorexia, Bulimia can also be accompanied by other mental illnesses, and it's common to find that the person is depressed, anxious or may be self-harming.

Awareness and warning signs

> *"We realised something was wrong when Rose started not
> wanting to eat meals with us. In the half-term holidays days out
> and family gatherings became difficult because she didn't want
> to participate in the things which involved food. She began to
> question the calories on every packet and if she saw that
> anything was 400 calories or over she went mad and refused to
> eat it." - Alison*

Because I was fourteen, I was at secondary school when I started to
become noticeably ill with Anorexia. It was easier for me to quickly lose
a lot of weight, because I'd tell my parents I was eating at school when
actually my lovingly-prepared lunch was going in the bin. In the evening I
hardly ate anything, blaming my poor appetite on having eating so much
though the day. My parents didn't suspect anything because I used to
eat such a lot, and they knew I was making a conscious effort to diet
because I was unhappy with my body.

It was only when I started to look gaunt and my clothes began to hang
off me that my parents (and others) started to worry that the weight
loss had gone 'too far.' But by then I was consumed with what I was
doing, rapidly becoming emaciated as I rationed my food intake to just a
couple of hundred calories and became suspicious and irritable as my
personality faded.

> *"We began to notice that Rose was exercising a lot. We could
> hear her banging about upstairs every single evening – the
> floorboards were creaking. One day I found her packed lunch
> untouched in her bag and I realised that she had been lying to
> us. That's when I knew for sure that something was wrong." –
> Alison*

Awareness and urgency are both key when it comes to fighting an eating disorder – so be vigilant and once you suspect that your child has an eating disorder, start to gather as much information as possible and consult with your GP to see which course of action you can take.

5. Why do people develop eating disorders?

Whenever anybody suffers with a debilitating, all-consuming physical or mental illness, the first question many people around them ask is 'Why'? Why this person?' Because eating disorders have devastating physical and mental consequences, it can be even harder for family members and friends to accept - especially because it is difficult for anybody without the illness to truly understand. I know from personal experience that misunderstanding (especially alongside anger) can make things worse for an individual with an eating disorder – but playing the 'blame game' is never helpful. Finding the root cause, however, can be useful – because this can help the person to identify the beliefs which have caused them to feel the way they do, and should go some way to aiding their recovery.

Everyone is different

The first thing to say when talking about causes and triggers behind an eating disorder is that everyone is different – so naturally from one person to the next the reason behind the illness will be different. It's difficult to be able to place the 'blame' for an eating disorder at the feet of one thing in particular, because it's often a combination of things which results in the illness rather than one issue alone. There are triggers –for example a traumatic life event such as the death of a loved one, or internal issues which build up over time as a consequence of bullying or sexual abuse. It might be that there's nothing blindingly obvious - just a feeling of discontentment which has been bubbling away for months or even years and slowly leads to the eating disorder. Eating disorders are also often accompanied by other mental illnesses - for example, I had OCD and Body Dysmorphic Disorder too. Others might have Bipolar Disorder, Depression or Anxiety. Recognising this can help people to understand how complex an illness this really is - especially when it does come along with other complications.

Media and culture DO have roles to play

I once read an article written by a top psychologist claiming that society's obsession with 'perfect' and in particular 'the perfect (slim) body' had absolutely nothing to do with the development of eating disorders, in particular Anorexia. As someone who went through Anorexia, I have to disagree.

I developed Anorexia for many different reasons - but the root for me was being bullied for being fat. I decided (with the help of the media and kids at school) that thin people were liked, and embarked upon a journey of fad dieting which ultimately led me to become completely obsessed and very poorly. Whilst my self-hatred, perfectionism and lack of control over my life certainly had a lot to do with my illness, with the correct nutritional advice, kindness and encouragement from the right sources I might have better understood how my body worked, respected it rather than hated it, and been able to see the world with a more rational perspective. I may have developed a healthier level of self-worth, maintained more positive mental wellbeing, lost the weight I needed to lose safely and with a new-found self-confidence I might not have cared so much about what people at school said about me. Instead I was influenced by celebrity magazines and dubious information from diet companies. I was taken in by adverts and TV programmes which showed me who I 'should be' and clearly highlighted who I was not and why I didn't fit in.

Pressure in today's society isn't purely aesthetic, either. Pressure to excel in every area of our lives is becoming a huge trigger for eating disorders, as is a life increasingly lived on and through a screen. We're exposed to other people's lives more than we ever have been before, and this in turn encourages us to compare, often unfavourably.

Perfectionism and control matter

I am naturally a perfectionist and I like to be in control. This is in part a personality trait, but also perhaps a product of what I have been through in life. Several studies have shown that people who have these personality traits can be predisposed to developing an eating disorder. People with OCD and generally obsessive or anxious personalities (like myself) can also be susceptible to eating disorders by nature.

Food ends up being the resulting behaviour - because food is easy for us to control. The root is self-loathing, a feeling of total lack of control, a desire to be 'perfect' and a strong determination to reach goals. And when goals are not reached, a punishing, critical voice inside which scrutinises everything which could have been improved upon and berates you internally. All of this in turn can of course affect how you behave externally. As above, it's different for everyone.

Statistics show that more and more people are developing eating disorders, at increasingly young ages. I think largely this is down to social pressure – now as adults and as children we are expected to be clever, good looking, funny, popular, interesting all at once – the list goes on. Society focuses on what we haven't got and places large amounts of value on material things without considering what's on the inside. Schools and colleges place huge academic pressure on children at early ages, with targets and grades and league tables taking precedence over the mental health of our young people. Bullying is more prevalent than ever before with an increased number of avenues for bullies to exploit, whilst social media encourages a culture of having more or 'needing' to have more.

Perfectionism has always been a part of me and certainly contributed to my development of Anorexia – but now, anything less than perfect is rarely acceptable. 'Perfect' is depicted as attainable by celebrities, social networks and other media, so naturally younger people feel pressure to be perfect, look perfect and have a 'perfect' life. Of course perfect doesn't exist, so many children and young people feel disappointed and ashamed when they don't live up to society's ideals. When surveyed, UK children were amongst the unhappiest in the world, coming 14th out of 15 countries including Ethiopia, Colombia and Romania for overall life satisfaction – and as external pressures, perfectionism and bullying were causes behind my own eating disorder I believe this statistic must be intrinsically linked to the rise in eating disorders amongst children, teens and younger people.

Whilst it might feel as though reading this now your child already has an eating disorder is pointless, it's important to know the possible root as then you can take care not to exacerbate the negative beliefs and feelings your child has around that particular part of themselves as they recover, and instead work to build them up where they need support. It's also key to know that an eating disorder is nobody's 'fault' – not yours, and not your child's. This will be covered I greater detail later.

6. Your role in recovery

As I say in the introduction, without my parents I don't believe I would be here today. I say that because it's very true – I was let down by the psychological and medical teams who were supposed to help me, and when they gave up I was discharged home even though mentally I was in a worse state than when I'd been admitted. If I had gone home to parents who weren't prepared to face the challenges of helping me through, who couldn't fight my battle for me whilst I was too weak to do so myself, I would still be poorly now, or I would have died.

I don't say these things to put pressure on you, or to make you feel as though this is a journey you must take alone. However it's important to be aware that whatever situation your child is in, your role in their recovery is an essential one.

Becoming a different parent

Your role as a parent is about to change. Whilst you are still the supportive, loving mum or dad you were before, you are also going to have to adopt a different persona in order to help your child through this. Dogged determination, perseverance and a degree of separation are needed, and this might require a change in your style of parenting compared with what you are used to.

Being strict

> *"Being strict was the hardest thing, really. Because it felt as though we were being hard on Rose, but we had to be in order to fight Anorexia." - John*

When I was in hospital another girl with Anorexia briefly stayed in the same ward as me. I had a lot of restrictions placed on me which meant my parents and other family members couldn't visit very often, so I spent a lot of time on my own (not that this was particularly good for me). In contrast, this girl's family were at her bedside 24/7. But they inadvertently did more harm than good. They were present at every mealtime to ensure that staff didn't force her to follow the diet plan she'd been given – on hand with diet yoghurts, low-carb bread and fat-free milk to replace the food on offer from the hospital. They went to the shops every single day to buy her the specific food she included on her shopping list – only whilst they believed were making *her* happy (and it certainly appeared that way), they were making her eating disorder happy – and literally killing her with kindness in the process.

Many parents find it hard to say 'no' to their child, especially when they are ill. But in this situation you are saying no to the eating disorder, which makes it more likely that your child will be healthy and well again. At the time, it seems like it's your child who is kicking you, screaming at you, crying and telling you they hate you. But it's not. It's like an exorcism – the good comes after the bad.

I would often do all of those things. But afterwards, even just for a brief second, I'd have a rational moment. Because the 'me' deep down knew that my parents would never do anything to hurt me – that they'd only do what was in my very best interests. Slowly but surely that belief grew stronger until eventually I knew that I should believe them when they said I should get better and that my life was worth living – and that it wouldn't be terrible if I gained weight and became physically healthy again, letting go of Anorexia. There's more about separating your child from their eating disorder in the next chapter.

Staying strong and looking after yourself

> "Even though it was hard, I made a conscious effort to eat and drink enough myself. It's so important to look after yourself, because there's a tendency to feel as though there's no light at the end of the tunnel." - Alison

Fighting an eating disorder is exhausting. It can be mentally and physically draining – especially if your child is at home constantly or is staying in a hospital which requires you to make a long journey to visit. That's why it's especially important that you take care of your own mental and physical wellbeing whilst you are going through this difficult time.

Make sure you have time to eat properly, and try to stay away from popular coping mechanisms such as alcohol. The healthier you are yourself, the more able you will be to help your child. Relationships can also become strained as a result of the stress involved in caring for a child with an eating disorder, so try to make quality time for your family (other children and partners or spouses) which doesn't involve discussing the eating disorder to try to maintain a sense of normality for everyone else involved. Whilst it might be difficult to enjoy activities with so much going on, it's likely that as individuals and as a family unit relationships will suffer if life begins to centre around the eating disorder at all times.

"I was open and honest with my employer and I also received counselling whilst I was supporting Rose through Anorexia. It was very difficult to be strong for her and have anything left for myself at the end of the day." – Alison

As my mum did, it's also a good idea to make sure that you inform your workplace about what is going on so that they can also support you and make allowances for you if you need them to.

Gathering as much support and advice as possible

"The best thing that I did was to open up to people around me that I felt I could trust. What you need is someone to sound off against, someone to talk about it to and talk things through with. You can't keep it to yourself because it's such a hard thing to do to be that strong, so you need people around you who you can talk to - a good support network." - Alison

You're already taking steps to gain more information and support just by reading this book. There are other resources online and forums which can help, as well as counselling services which can offer you an impartial person to bounce off when things get too much. But support can come from other places, too. If you are able to, call on family and friends to help you out. They don't have to be directly involved – just small things like taking care of other children or doing some washing could make a real difference when you are juggling a job and multiple hospital visits or are having to watch your child all the time. If you don't have anyone you can ask, look into volunteer groups and charities who may be able to point you in the direction of organisations who can help.

7. Separating your child from their eating disorder

"Always remember it isn't your child that's screaming and shouting – it is the illness, and you have to be able to almost switch off and spot the difference, to separate the two, because that gives you the strength to fight the illness and stops you from feeling so guilty. It's still very difficult, but it's impossible if you don't get your head around that." – Alison

Many people with an eating disorder (Anorexia, especially) find themselves at the centre of blame for their condition - mostly because of a lack of understanding at best and ignorance at worse. I encountered so many people who believed that I was poorly by choice - and therefore thought I deserved what I got because I was being deliberately obstinate. I think this is true of many mental illnesses - because it's hard for people on the outside to differentiate between the person inside and the 'demon' alongside them which forces them to behave out of character.

Earlier in this book and in Tough Cookie I describe Anorexia as a demonic entity - because it's the best way I can truly relate how it feels to suffer, but also to help people supporting someone who is suffering to differentiate between the two 'people' inside their loved one's head. If you can do this and effectively support and nourish the person left inside, then slowly the Anorexia will wither away as it lacks negatives to feed from.

Knowing what's your child, and what's the eating disorder

The problem many people have with psychological illnesses such as personality disorders and schizophrenia is that they don't know who they're talking to at any given time. Often they're unsure whether the words that come out of that person's mouth and their actions and behaviours are their own, or those of another person or entity.

I believe it's the same with an eating disorder. Eating disorders cause you to behave completely out of character – to do things you would never, ever do. They consume pieces of you until you have little personality left inside – but the 'real' you is in there somewhere, and you just need the will to fight out.

I am a very honest person and I was brought up to never, ever lie. But Anorexia is secretive and devious, and lying is part and parcel of reaching its end goal. At first it broke my heart to waste food and lie to my parents, but it also felt good. The good feeling didn't come from within me – it came from Anorexia. I became a different person – I was unrecognisable from the relatively healthy teenager I'd been before, and a thousand miles away from the happy, carefree child I'd been before I was bullied. Later on when I would sit on my bed and stare into space, devoid of any emotion or feeling, writing nasty things about people around me and meticulously logging any food and exercise in my diary. Manically researching calories and suspiciously Googling whether water contained any fat. When I watched my mum cry as she felt helpless after I'd thrown another plate of food on the floor. As I screamed and swore and threw myself around over a meal she'd spent ages preparing for me and desperately wanted me to eat. When my dad made a special journey to pick up something I used to love to eat and I threw it back in his face. None of it was me.

I think the mistake a lot of families make is that they assume that the person themselves is being unreasonable and has changed into someone they don't recognise, which then makes them a lot harder to deal with. It also makes it easier to say cruel things and make throwaway comments in the heat of the moment in an attempt to get the person to listen, such as 'You're doing this to spite us', 'Look how upset you're making your mum', 'You're not even trying to eat' 'Are you stupid?' and so on.

I believe that the key to fighting an eating disorder and supporting someone through recovery is understanding the way an eating disorder works, and getting to know it intimately so that you can more easily spot which behaviours belong to your child, and which don't. Once you're able to split them you can then set about fighting the eating disorder, whilst nurturing your child and giving them the much-needed support and care they need mentally to get through this.

My parents largely did this without knowing it. Whilst they were firm and strong about food and at mealtimes, withstanding the hurling and the screaming and shouting, they planned things for me so that I slowly began to feel I could be in love with my life again. I liked to be outside, so they'd hire a wheelchair for me and we'd go for walks in the sun. Mum would make CDs of my favourite music and we'd go for a run out in the car. They'd take me to the garden centre to see the animals. All of these things were positive distractions, but equally they showed me that I was still cared for and loved despite everything, and proved that there were other things I enjoyed besides controlling food. Eventually I decided I wanted to live, and I was strong enough to resolve to fight Anorexia. Although it was still there within me and the hard work for me had only just begun, the point was that the 'me' inside had decided I didn't want to share my space with this demon any longer.

When people say a person 'isn't ready to recover' or 'doesn't want to get better', it's simply because they are not supported enough in the right way to feel as though they want to listen to anything other than the negative dialogue their eating disorder has placed in their head. Eating disorders are cunning and cruel – and they rob you of all the things you loved and any passion or joy, leaving you devoid of emotion and personality. The only time I felt any excitement was when I was limiting my food, and even then that diminished as I started eating and drinking next to nothing, as there was nothing to count. As you reach a very low weight, your body begins to shut down, but your brain is also starved. It is harder to think rationally, to make sound decisions, or to understand the words and actions of other people. You're weak, exhausted and just consumed by the thoughts the eating disorder has planted in your head – believing fully that this is what you deserve, that you're doing the right thing, there's no other way – everyone else is wrong or lying. This is also important to bear in mind when you're dealing with your child (and not the eating disorder).

I know that recognising and nurturing the person left inside so that they feel able and aren't frightened of starting to fight their eating disorder is key to recovery – because that's how I overcame Anorexia. Inadvertently my parents were tough enough when it counted, but made a massive effort to instil hope and happiness back into the 'me' left inside.

Whenever you're thinking of getting angry or feel frustrated with your child, remember to try and recognise whether what they are saying or doing is a product of their personality. If not, handle it appropriately. If they're desperately asking for help, assume your role as a caring parent and love them as you always have done. In 'What to do, and what not to do' I discuss in further detail the positive things which helped me to get to a point mentally where I felt I wanted to fight my eating disorder, and examples of things you can do too.

Guilt

I discuss guilt in more detail later on in the book, but it does have a place at the end of this chapter, too. That's because inadvertently, you can cause your child to feel guilty when they feel powerless to change their behaviour. They're still not strong enough to want to fight, yet they feel terribly guilty about how they are making you feel and the impact their illness is having on your lives. Although I understand that in the heat of the moment you can say things you don't mean, try to be careful with what you say and do – because both in the short- and long-term, blaming your child or highlighting to them how their illness has had a negative impact on a loved one or the family as a whole is going to be harmful.

8. What is helpful, and what's not

"It's always so hard to know whether you are doing the right thing. Luckily we had some support from a therapist who told us what we needed to say and do to help Rose. She also told us the things which could exacerbate the situation or make things worse for her, so we felt more confident in how we handled the trickiest times, like mealtimes, and knew we were doing the right thing when we made time for her and did other things to positively help her recovery." – John

As a parent of a child with an eating disorder, there may always be a fear in the back of your mind that you will 'make things worse'. Even little things you do and say come under self-scrutiny, and you worry that your child may not recover or will come to hate you because you are going against what they appear to want to do. You may also find that other people - family members, colleagues, friends and even health professionals - inadvertently or deliberately cause you to feel bad about how you are handling the situation.

Many parents say they feel helpless and confused, worried that everything they do and say is making things worse without a solid understanding of what they can do to make things better. I start with what *isn't* helpful, because in lots of ways, I think it's more important to know what *not* to do first so that you can then understand why an alternative approach is more helpful and beneficial. If you read this section and find you've been approaching the situation 'all wrong', then don't worry – it's not too late to change.

What isn't helpful?

Lack of urgency

The biggest first step is recognising and admitting you have a problem, and then asking for help, so if your child is at this stage, support them as much as you possibly can by telling them that you are there for them, you'll help them through this, and gathering as much information and as many resources as you feel you need. Contact your GP or local hospital immediately and be perseverant and determined – don't take no for an answer and if you struggle to be listened to, keep trying, or go elsewhere.

Each week and each day that goes by is critical with an eating disorder. Day by day you lose more weight, become weaker, more poorly. Delays and denial of access to services *feeds* the eating disorder. It can make you feel helpless and frustrated if you find you can't access the help you need, so if you can't get the support you need there are other organisations (such as Tough Cookie) and charities who may be able to advise and guide you.

Blame

Whenever something 'bad' happens, it's human nature to want someone or something to blame. But playing the blame game where eating disorders are concerned is a dangerous and potentially harmful tactic.

Blame can be centred around you, or it can be centred on your child – or both of you. Either way, it only serves to make you feel bad at a time when you both need to feel as strong as possible. Perhaps family members, colleagues or friends are pointing the finger because you are recently divorced, or went on a diet. Maybe they say your child was always 'weak' or 'sensitive' or 'stubborn'. Wherever the misplaced blame is directed, it's not helpful – so it's best to shut it down and politely tell the person in question that you don't appreciate their comments.

My mum had just lost her dad (and I had lost my Grandad) not long before I started to become poorly. The person who later became my therapist at CAMHS called her and proceeded to berate her for not having accessed the service sooner – apparently unaware that my mum had been trying to get me the help I needed for *months*. My mum still feels guilty as a result and I could never forgive him for hurting one of the people I love the most – a person who gave me a lot more psychological and emotional support than they did!

An eating disorder (and the progression of an eating disorder) isn't anybody's 'fault'. If I was looking for someone to blame then I'd have to point the finger at my school and the people who bullied me, but that doesn't solve anything. Whilst identifying a cause is important, going over past events and trying to find an individual to blame is fruitless and can actually be quite harmful for everyone involved.

Frustration and anger

It's very easy to become frustrated with a child with an eating disorder. I know my parents did often – and speaking to others I regularly hear that family members lose their rag and say hurtful things. I think this is because (forgivably) they forget momentarily that the eating disorder is not the person standing in front of them, so they lash out at the eating disorder, but of course the person on the receiving end is the child.

I don't expect for a second that parents should always maintain a calm, sensitive demeanour and should never, ever lash out or say things they don't mean – that's inevitable. But being aware that constant anger and frustration can be damaging and can impede recovery is important.

One girl I spoke to told me that her Dad refused to come and see her in hospital. He said that was because he was 'sick of her not making an effort' and 'fed up of her being stupid' – he said he couldn't cope. This is a classic example of personal frustration and anger clouding judgement and ultimately hurting the child at the centre of the situation, because really they need as much support as possible and will suffer more if they feel that they are upsetting or angering you.

Ignorance and misunderstanding

I've already discussed how misconceptions can be harmful – which is why I de-bunked them earlier to hopefully prevent them from harming your child's chances of recovery. But sometimes, ignorance can come in a more innocent form which can be just as harmful for your child and their recovery.

I've discussed in some detail how Anorexia works in secretive, cunning ways – and some of that information may have surprised you. The reason I included it was to share for anyone who hasn't come into contact with an eating disorder just how devious they can be – however lovely and trustworthy the person suffering may be. They're not the ones in control – even though it appears that way.

Anorexia is cunning and clever. You cannot ever underestimate the lengths it will go to stop food and water going into your mouth. It will

42

hurt your family and friends and see you dead before it stops getting its own way and that is the unfortunate seriousness of this mental illness.

Because I wasn't watched enough by innocent staff, I continued to do a lot of exercise during my stay in hospital and I was able to squirrel all that food away. I don't think that this was actually neglectful – I think they trusted me and didn't have any understanding of Anorexia which would have made them suspicious or more careful. My parents however were much more vigilant. They had to adopt a 'zero tolerance, zero trust' approach – which was unpleasant for me at the time, but enabled them slowly to ensure that I was eating a little more - as a result I became more rational and open to their suggestions and support.

Negativity

I can't stress enough how important it is to be careful with your dialogue and to think about what you say to your child – and what it means to them. Even when you think you are being helpful or well-meaning, your words can inadvertently translate into something entirely different in their head – as I've mentioned when talking about the things people do and say which they believe to be useful ('just eat', for example).

Whilst you're bound to become angry and frustrated as I say above, if you tell them they'll 'never recover unless they start to change' or 'will die if they carry on' they'll believe it - and they will inevitably feel bad about themselves. My self-esteem and sense of self-worth was at an all-time low during my time with Anorexia, so I took every criticism to heart and genuinely believed that when people berated me for being poorly, it meant they didn't want me around and that it would be better for everyone involved if I did die after all. Meanwhile, Anorexia used these type of comments to feed off – 'see, you might as well die', 'you'd be better off dead'.

For this reason it's crucial that you try and keep all dialogue between you and your child as positive as possible, and avoid using accusative phrases or words 'selfish', 'stupid', and 'inconsiderate'. Additionally referring to death or the lasting effect of an eating disorder ('all your teeth will fall out', 'you won't be able to have children') is only going to make things much worse for your child, not better – as these 'threats' only feed the eating disorder and make your child weaker because they feel guilty and fearful. However much you want them to, it's unlikely they'll suddenly 'snap out of it', especially when they are listening to a constant stream of negative dialogue and their self-worth is battered by guilty thoughts.

We know how easy it is for the words and opinions of others to form inner belief and internal dialogues within ourselves – just as the words of my bullies caused me to believe I was ugly and worthless.

Telling someone with Anorexia to 'just eat' or a person with Bulimia not to make themselves sick implies that it is as simple as putting food in your mouth, assuming you have control. Saying 'you don't have a choice so you might as well just do it' and 'you're not trying' is aggressive and hurtful, and is as useful as telling somebody with a broken leg to 'fix it themselves'. Please don't tell someone to 'just eat' or that they're not trying hard enough to recover – they're not in control.

What _is_ helpful?

This is equally if not more important than talking about the things which are harmful and damaging – because these are the things that can help and increase the chances of eventually eliminating Anorexia for good.

Kindness and consideration – nurture the person inside

Compassion is key when it comes to eating disorders. I think that's because as I've said, whilst you present as somebody who isn't you, _you_ are still there inside somewhere and you need kindness more than ever. Unfortunately an eating disorder needs harsh firm treatment and being separated from it doesn't at all feel good because you are so absorbed in all the cruel lies it's told you about yourself and about your life. Eventually, though, it is possible and you _can_ squash that voice in your head.

To do this, I believe a balance is needed. A balance of targeted therapy and medical treatment which does involve a firm, uncompromising approach and careful rediscovery of the personality, dreams and hope that may have been lost along the way through kindness and empathy.

Don't make assumptions - even if you don't understand. Instead make a point of being generous and friendly. Nurture the person inside. Remember that they are not the eating disorder, and the eating disorder is not them.

The truth is, overcoming an eating disorder is down to the individual. The responsibility lies with them; and only them. It's not something you can force them to do.

At the moment, they don't feel like life is worth living. That may not be something you feel able to change, but there are things that you can do to help them believe they are worthy of life just as anyone else is, and that they are capable and deserving of recovering and doing the things they want to.

Everyone has dreams. Likes, dislikes. We're all passionate about something. An eating disorder makes you passionate about only one thing: controlling food. It supresses all the other things you loved doing and replaces your life with one which revolves around disappearing, physically and psychologically. But that person you love is still in there somewhere! They still want to do the things they always did. They have a warped perception of reality at the moment, and food will still be getting in the way of their dreams and day to day life. I still had dreams, (I wanted to live abroad by the beach) but in my dreams I lived off one cereal bar a day (which was perfectly acceptable to my completely irrational mind), and I weighed 6 stone (a massive 1.5 stone increase from where I was at the time, which seemed like a colossal amount to me at that point).

Treatment of Anorexia has to feel harsh and unpleasant to be effective. It's going to hurt the sufferer by default, because they wholly believe that what they are thinking is a product of their own mind and not a mental illness. This is why I think it's really important to show kindness too, whilst showing the eating disorder absolutely no mercy.

The difficulty for parents and professionals alike is that you care about that person's health and want them to be happy. But it's hard to decipher whether what they are telling you will make them happy or whether it actually makes the eating disorder happy and therefore contributes to their illness. Generally, what they say makes them happy is not what makes them healthy. Remember that it isn't them – it is the illness, and that there is still a person in there who has things (unrelated to food and exercise) which make them happy. Focus on these. Find, feed and encourage things that make that person happy which are completely unrelated to the eating disorder. For me, that was getting a pet, going for a walk, having a look round the garden centre.

By likening Anorexia to a demon I am not waiving responsibility for how I behaved and what I put my family through. However I think it's important to separate the two when you look at someone you love who is suffering. Nurture the person inside them who is lost and screaming to get out – show the eating disorder no mercy, yet give the person left love and attention. They are already at their lowest ebb, feeling helpless and worthless and guilty. By showing them they have something to live for, sharing their favourite activities with them, and encouraging them to look forward to the future, you help them grow and grow until eventually the demon inside their head grows smaller and smaller.

Whilst they are crying over the prospect of eating a meal, promise something fun at the end of it. Spend time with them, encourage them to spend time on themselves such as having a manicure or hand massage. One health worker Mary used to come and give me a manicure and hand massage every week; she brought in nail polish, olive oil and hand cream just so that she could do that for me. One nurse, Joy, used to take me around the hospital grounds in my wheelchair and sit out in the sun with me. Joy always mentioned my smile and never the rest of me. She gave me hugs and genuinely wanted me to be well again. We would talk about the future, my plans, where I wanted to live and what I wanted to do. She always told me I had a beautiful smile; she was such a kind, positive, happy lady. These people made me feel like I was worth talking to and spending time with, whilst most other health professionals avoided me. They were angry and frustrated with me; they thought of me as a time waster. Of course my parents were incredible too – and as I say throughout this book, I credit them alone with my recovery. They would take me out for long wheelchair rides in the evenings too when they were allowed to visit, and when I was able to they would do lots of nice things with me so that slowly, I remembered who I was and why I was living. I remember those people and what they did for me so strongly and I am so thankful for their kindness and patience. The simple things they did made a huge difference and aided my complete recovery.

So you can see, you can make a huge difference to your child simply by being kind – even when you don't feel like it because you're exhausted, or angry because you've just had a screaming match over a meal. The smallest things had the biggest impacts – going shopping with my family my cousin making me do wheelies in the wheelchair – driving out in the evening sun listening to music. Being in nature, sitting with the sun on my face with Joy as we talked about the future.

I'm not a psychologist - I only speak from experience. But I believe that showing kindness whilst having to treat a mental illness so harshly and urgently is essential for the recovery of that person.

Helping and encouraging your child to focus on something positive

In Tough Cookie I talk about one of the biggest catalysts for recovery being an ability to picture the future and look forward to positive things coming up, as well as identifying the good things in life right now. When you have an eating disorder it can be hard for you to do this all by yourself, especially if you are consumed by a negative mind-set.

So it's really helpful for family, friends and carers to lend a helping hand. Make them feel important inside – encourage them to talk about what they like what they have to live for and give them practical examples of how they can start to do that right now. Look through magazines and at visual aids with them to make the goals tangible. More than anything this gives them hope indirectly without seeming like a conscious effort to combat the eating disorder.

You can discover incredible things about yourself – what you want, what you're capable of and things you really enjoy when you have eating disorder. And just like any serious illness, having a near miss like that can make you really appreciate your life. Many incredible artists, writers and musicians emerged from the face of adversity.

Joy encouraged me to talk about the future and what I wanted in my life. She'd take me out in my wheelchair and we'd sit in a spot on the hospital grounds in the warm sun. She asked me what I was going to do when I was 'better'. Coming from her, I didn't see it as a loaded question or a trick – I saw that she was genuinely interested and cared about me. Together, we laid exciting plans for my life abroad by the sea. I'd talk excitedly about them to my parents who helped me to elaborate on my vision until it was looking grand and too good to forget or ignore. I still have those dreams today – and although I didn't know it at the time looking back I know that focusing on things like that helped me to want to recover.

I include visualisation tools and brainstorms in Tough Cookie which are easy to fill out and can help to fire up the person left inside by identifying what it is they truly desire – and realising that they can't have those things whilst they're still consumed by Anorexia.

I knew I couldn't have those things and Anorexia simultaneously – something would have to give. And inside those things made me feel good, but Anorexia invariably made me feel bad.

Recognise signs of recovery and encourage and support

Recognising and noticing the early indications that your child is starting to feel like they want to get better is really important. You can then encourage them and give them the support they will need to continue feeling strong enough to recover. People tend to talk about recovery as though it's a straight, steady upward road when you reach the top and you're 'better'. But actually it can be a long, hard slog filled with peaks and troughs and though there will be lots of good days and positive progress there might also be setbacks and relapses.

Initial signs of recovery are subtle but if you know what to look out for they're not too difficult to spot. When I had Anorexia, I had completely lost my personality. I spent most of the time silently staring into space – I only became animated if I was threatened with the prospect of having to food. Any tiny spark of my personality in the midst of the way I presented whilst I was consumed with Anorexia was a sign of the 'me' inside showing through. Showing interest in things other than food or eating – talking about the future, laughing or even smiling at a joke. These are all things to look out for.

I also say in Tough Cookie that for me, guilt was one of the first signs that I was getting stronger. Anorexia is so powerful that it almost shuts out the guilt when you are throwing away a lovingly prepared meal or screaming at your loved ones. Feeling any element of guilt was certainly for me a turning point. Although at first it wasn't pleasant to feel so guilty but also feeling so helpless to do anything about hurting the people I loved, it was part of the recovery process.

With zero respect or love for myself (and no therapy to help me to change that), I recovered for the sake of my parents. We're always

50

encouraged to do things for ourselves and only us, and that's undeniably true. In an ideal world, that's what would happen. But how many of us really do things for ourselves? We tend to have more love in our hearts for others than we do for ourselves. I think it's important recognise that people's motive for recovery might not be 'healthy' or 'ideal'; but if it's a motive it's a motive – let it be and once they are on their way they will be more responsive to therapy, more open to perhaps feeling better about themselves and that *they* are worth a healthy, happy life. The motive isn't so important – what is crucial is that that person feels ready to make a change and live their lives - and whatever the circumstances that should be encouraged.

Supporting each other and looking after yourself

Watching your loved one turn into someone you don't recognise – physically and personality-wise is an upsetting experience that simply cannot be trivialised. You've lost the person you thought you knew – and desperately want them back.

My parents have always said they couldn't have helped me without the support of a therapist they had at the hospital who was actually very generous and caring. She gave them the tools and advice and listened to them when they became dejected and downhearted if I wasn't doing too well. Recovery is a struggle – and more and more families are dealing with Anorexia alone because of a lack of places on specialist wards.

The pressure on you at the moment as a parent, carer or friend is enormous. You may feel responsible for this person and their recovery.

It's the hardest thing in the world to helplessly watch someone you love slowly killing themselves, feeling powerless to do anything about it.

One thing I've noticed when speaking to parents is that the ones who try to take care of themselves and support their families have stronger, more resilient children as a result. For me it's so important for parents and family members to understand what to do and what not to do in such a distressing and confusing time, especially when there's often little support for families who are going through it with their loved ones. Whilst the experience was traumatic for me, I was so wrapped up in my own suffering that I think it was actually harder on my parents, who were fully present and so had to witness my self-destruction and had to struggle and fight for my survival and recovery – and with me having no help or support from anyone else, that made it a million times harder for them. The dynamics in our house were very strange, because my parents naturally (like most parents) wanted to feed me and see me happy and healthy. Of course I understood that deep down, and to know you are hurting your loved ones but feeling powerless to do anything about it is horrendous. Only now I fully appreciate the fact that they worked as a team and tried hard not to make me feel guilty or punish me.

I'm not saying they always got it right, but in the end, they succeeded.

> *"Even with the knowledge and support we were given we didn't always get it right. Nobody can. We still made mistakes and I often got to the point where I was so desperate and upset that I would plead and beg Rose to eat, but that didn't make any difference because we both just ended up sad and arguing or feeling helpless and guilty." – Alison*

Luckily, they had access to the therapist who had gone out of her way to research Anorexia and armed with a few tools helped them to get through it and get me through it, too. Not all parents have access to that kind of support – but as I say frequently in this book, even small things make a difference. Perhaps you can look into accessing a counselling service, or a book you could read – maybe you have heard about support groups or forums where you can speak to other parents in the same position. Try to remember that you are going through something tough, and you doing really well to keep everything together.

9. Helping others to understand an eating disorder

"One of the most difficult things was helping family members and friends to understand that it's a mental illness and she couldn't just 'snap out of it' or 'start eating' – she wasn't doing it on purpose. Trying to explain that over and over again felt impossible at times." – Alison

One of the things which made my life more difficult whilst I recovered from Anorexia were the reactions and treatment I received from people around me. From family and so-called friends to strangers in the street and the nurses and staff who were supposed to be looking after me, I was met with mixed reception and often attacked personally for being the way I was. People stared at me and whispered about me. It didn't occur to many people that Anorexia wasn't a choice. It is a very difficult thing for people to get their heads around – which is why I do what I do with a goal of using my own experience to explain Anorexia to others. I hope that the initial explanations in this book have helped you to understand eating disorders in more detail – but once you understand, how do you help others to do the same?

Explain that an eating disorder is not a choice

Just as I did at the start of this book, this is the first and most important thing to explain to a family member or friend – that an eating disorder is an illness, just like a physical illness, and therefore, choice doesn't really come into it. Grandparents and older generations especially can be scathing about mental illness in general, but especially eating disorders such as Anorexia and Bulimia – because food is such a huge element in our lives. Every time a family meal comes around or a visit (accompanied by tea and biscuits), your child's illness is starkly emphasised and becomes an issue. Even my teachers and nurses in hospital implied that I was being awkward and obstinate – that I should stop being so bloody stubborn and 'just eat'. Yes, as an individual a person with an eating disorder has the power and responsibility to recover – nobody can do it for them. But they need support and help to get there – and what they don't need is people telling them to 'stop'.

Explain that an eating disorder is about more than just food

As you will know having read previous chapters, another common misconception about eating disorders is that they are all about food. Because it manifests itself in the form of an extreme diet and fitness regime resulting in dramatic weight loss, most people assume that the person is image obsessed and overly concerned with their weight. But this is a symptom, not necessarily a cause (although in my case, I was influenced by these things). An eating disorder has many possible causes as you will have read previously – and it is often accompanied by other mental illnesses (depression, self-harm, OCD). To simplify it for a person who doesn't understand, explain that it is a form of self-hatred and a need for control which is not just appearance-related. Perfectionism and a feeling of inadequacy are often behind eating disorders, along with traumatic family events and a loss of control over life such as death or unemployment. Be prepared for people to assume otherwise and not wish to consider that there might be more to it than meets the eye.

Explain that there are two entities in your child's head

Use my analogy of a demonic entity that needs exorcising to help the person separate your child away from their behaviour. Explain that your child needs love and encouragement, but emphasise that at the same time the eating disorder needs showing where to go. That's why your behaviour and the way you handle them might seem strange. People might start telling you what to do: 'well, I wouldn't have done it like that' or 'you're letting them get away with it' or 'you're being too harsh.' Unless that person is a specialist medical professional or psychiatrist experienced in eating disorders, *take no notice*.

Explain that guilt and blame are not helpful

If a family member starts berating your child for 'not eating' or highlighting the effect that 'what they are doing' is having on the family as a whole, then please stop them and explain that this will make things worse. Just because a person with an eating disorder continues with what they are doing helplessly, it does not mean they are not feeling guilty. They think they are in control, but they're not. They can hear the things you are saying to them and deep down inside they may want to be 'normal' and to stop but they just don't feel able to. They are not poorly on purpose and they're certainly not making a choice to behave in this way – as explained above. It's as bad as blaming someone with cancer for having cancer – so once again use this analogy if you have to and explain that an eating disorder is an illness, not a choice.

10. Finding help and support

One of the biggest things you hear in the press about eating disorders (and indeed when I speak to sufferers and their parents, GPs and other professionals) is the lack of support available to people with eating disorders in the UK – especially those under the age of 16 – and how hard it is to be listened to and taken seriously. There was pretty much nothing for me when I was poorly – but a decade on, things have improved. This chapter should give you an idea of what to expect when you ask for help, and what you can do if you find you can't access the support you need.

Speaking with your GP

The first step for any parent who suspects their child may be suffering with an eating disorder is to visit the GP. Make an appointment alone if you are concerned about confronting your child, and explain the symptoms and situation with them informally before taking things further. Your GP should firstly be able to give you an idea of what's available in your area, and how the pathway works (i.e, what needs to happen and when, and what they can do depending on what condition your child is in). They can also offer advice and support for you as a parent and can point you in the direction of local groups and clinics. It's likely that if you do go alone first they will want to see your child to assess them fully (which may involve weighing them, taking bloods and checking BMI). They will then make a decision on the type of care and treatment they'll need.

Unfortunately with services stretched GPs aren't always able to refer owing to strict criteria – however much they want to. Instead, they may direct you to other organisations for help in the interim. My GP was excellent and she was very concerned even on our first visit – she knew something was wrong. But her hands were tied – she had nowhere to send me and CAMHS wouldn't intervene until things were critical. Don't lose heart or get angry if your GP is unable or unwilling to help – you are always entitled to a second opinion and other assistance is available.

What can I expect when I ask for help?

The NHS has a pathway for young people with eating disorders which starts with your visit to the GP. The level of support available and the quality of the provision may greatly differ from place to place and will depend on where you live and what's on offer in your Primary Care Trust. Following the initial visit you may be referred on to CAMHS (Child and Adolescent Mental Health Services), depending on the severity of your child's condition. CAMHS should fully assess your child and will be able to diagnose an eating disorder. They should then offer targeted therapy (which may include Cognitive Behavioural Therapy and Dialectical Behavioural Therapy) to help ascertain the root and causes and may involve other professionals such as dieticians to take care of the physical symptoms of the eating disorder. If this is not enough or your child is very poorly they may be admitted to a specialist EDU (Eating Disorder Unit) for young people with Anorexia or Bulimia (these are sometimes run by private healthcare companies, such as Priory).

I often talk openly about my negative experience with CAMHS and with my local hospital and work to improve services as much as I can. But that doesn't mean that your experience will be negative. This is partly why I'm passionate about sharing my story to prove that even if you feel you have been let down there are other things you can do.

Going further for help and support

If you don't feel that you are listened to, or you are being told that there is nothing available to you because you child isn't unwell enough, then there are other places where you may be able to access help and support. The frustrating thing about the way eating disorders (and indeed many serious mental health conditions) are handled in the UK is the lack of urgency – but often this can really make things worse for the person and allows the eating disorder to exacerbate with no support in place.

If you find you are not being listened to or haven't had a good experience at any level, it's important that you don't lose sight of the end goal, which is to help your child to be well again.

When my GP was unable to refer me my mum made a list of the available charities at the time and called them all to see if there was anything they could do. A lot of them were unable to help because of my age, but others did offer some advice which at least made my mum feel as though she was making some progress.

Now there are many more charities and a greater number of online resources, plus private practitioners who can help in the interim if you have funds available. You are not alone – and just by reading this book, you are taking an important step.

There are links at the back of this book which contain details of some helpful charities and organisations including my own, Tough Cookie.

11. Recovery – what now?

It would be impossible for me to talk about every element of recovery in this book, because it's different for everyone, and it can be a long and complex process filled with ups and downs. What I can do however is to talk about how I experienced recovery, how my parents were an important part of that and how we rebuilt our lives after what happened.

Maintain a positive relationship with food

I can't stress this enough. Part of the work I do with men and women of all ages, but especially with young people, is showing them that a positive relationship with food is the only way to live happily and healthily. To have a good relationship with your body and to feel as though you don't need to control it all the time, you need to let go of the misconceptions and myths we've all come to believe as a society after years of confusing advice from diet companies and food manufacturers.

Even once your child has recovered from their eating disorder, they may still have a distorted view of food – because let's face it, how many people *really* see food in a positive way? How many of us are confused or stressed about what we eat, how we eat, when we eat?

As a parent, showing an obsession with food and calories or condoning only eating certain things is never going to be good for a child who has experienced Anorexia or Bulimia. Instead, lead by example and don't make food a 'big thing' in your lives. Condone healthy, wholesome meals and never refer to the fat contained, or the calories, or the carbs. If you are on a diet yourself (diets are something I strongly disagree with) or want to enforce a healthy eating plan on other members of your family, do so discreetly. The best scenario, however, is for you all to be on the same page – with food as an important yet positive element of your life which doesn't hold any control over you.

You can find more about nutrition and a healthier relationship with food in my book, *Nutrition in a Nutshell.*

Keep working on strength, resilience and positive self-esteem

It's likely your child will continue to have therapy for a while after they become a 'healthy' weight – or at least they should if it is offered to them. That's because the belief systems behind eating disorders are often strong, and without proper treatment, they may cause further problems or a relapse down the line as deep down they are still present. Whilst I didn't ever relapse, I went on to develop other issues and the reason for this was that I never received proper psychological support during and after my eating disorder, so my intensely negative beliefs went untouched and were allowed to exacerbate. I was sensitive and guilty and went back to a school where I had been (and continued to be) bullied.

It's important to recognise that the triggers, causes and beliefs behind your child's eating disorder may not have gone away – sometimes, it's impossible to change that (for example, I could have moved schools, but I might have been bullied again, and the change would have been stressful for me). The most important thing you can do is to help your child build their resilience and deal with any adversity in a positive way, helping to reinforce positive beliefs rather than adding substance to the negative ones. By helping your child in challenging their negative beliefs you are helping to make them stronger mentally and less likely to relapse.

Use this experience to your advantage and enjoy the time that you have

Even though we've always been a closely-knit family, going through Anorexia brought us much closer together as a unit, and gave us a real appreciation of each other that you only find when you've been close to losing someone you love, but were given a second chance.

Try to enjoy the time you have and recognise when arguments are trivial or you're giving time to things which really don't matter.

Notice and be aware of signs of relapse, but don't be overly suspicious

One thing that *even now* I find difficult is the suspicion which I sometimes get from my family – a residual effect which is still lingering now over ten years since my eating disorder. I developed Irritable Bowel Syndrome around four years ago as a result of an anxiety disorder – and this means that sometimes it's hard for me to eat. Even when I am not particularly bad, there are things I'm not able to eat because they upset my stomach. This all sounds like an elaborate excuse someone with Anorexia might use (and indeed, I tried every trick in the book, including becoming 'vegan', when I was poorly), but in my case it's true. So when family members are impolite or exasperated, make comments about me being 'stubborn' or flash me disgruntled looks across the table at mealtimes, it's very frustrating. Firstly because if I did have an eating disorder, that would be the wrong way to deal with it, but secondly because I have a physical health problem and just want to mind my own business – I haven't had Anorexia for over a decade.

Being under scrutiny 24/7 is hard – especially if you've already been through an eating disorder and have been under constant monitoring and observation – something which isn't comfortable for any human being. Additionally, you should never use Anorexia as an insult. Even now I hear people say 'oh, she looks Anorexic' or 'He's so thin, he's Anorexic' to describe very thin people, when really they have no knowledge of that person's mental health or clinical status. They might have cancer, or be naturally very thin. Using Anorexia as an insult isn't nice for the person you aim it at, but it's also insulting for people like me who have been through it. It's not just about being thin, as you will know by now.

It's important to be vigilant and on guard to spot when your child's behaviour might be slightly unusual or concerning, but at the same time, try not to breathe down their neck or question them over every little thing. Whilst you might think that you are just doing your job as a parent, they will take it as an attack or an indication that you don't trust them or think they're not strong enough to keep going on their own without relapse. Keep supporting them and promoting positive mental wellbeing, reminding them of all the exciting things they have ahead of them in the future.

Withdrawing and reducing observation

> *'We found it very difficult to trust Rose for a long time. If she exercised or said she didn't want to eat something for whatever reason, even years afterwards, we'd get that pang of anxiety and think: is this it again?' - John*

Recognising which behaviours belong to your child and which don't allows you to be suspicious and distrusting of the eating disorder which is what it needs – constant observation and vigilance. But what happens when your child largely seems 'themselves' again? How do you spot the signs of relapse? How do you make sure it doesn't happen again? These are all real worries during and following recovery for parents, worries which manifest themselves in mistrust and cautious behaviour.

Constant observation comes with the territory of an eating disorder – but it can feel (both for you and your child) as though you're constantly on their back.

Eventually you will need to gradually reduce the level of observation and monitoring you have over your child. This can feel difficult, because there is always the spectre of relapse looming in the background. That's why withdrawing observation should be slow and subtle – your child shouldn't be able to detect that you are still keeping tabs on them and are carefully watching their behaviour so that they feel that you trust them, but at the same time, you still feel that you are in control and fully aware, taking no chances.

On both sides, integrity and authenticity is key, and an open and honest dialogue is also important. If you feel your child has been dishonest, don't approach them angrily or defensively. Instead try to talk about it calmly without an accusatory undertone – this way if you are right they are more likely to be responsive when you suggest that you need to support them more, and if you're wrong, they won't feel as though you don't trust them – as then the cycle of bad feeling begins again.

Regaining Trust

The only way to properly carry out the above withdrawal is to regain trust. I talk about regaining trust from a person with an eating disorder's perspective in Tough Cookie, explaining how they can show that their behaviour is honest and helping to build an important part of a relationship which has likely been broken down over the course of the illness. When you regain trust, you feel more able to withdraw observation completely.

Even once observation has been reduced dramatically, suspicion can still cause relations to be strained between you and your child as the try to stand on their own two feet again and rebuild their life.

I talk in Tough Cookie about regaining trust, and how for someone with an eating disorder, it can be hard to be trusted again following such a long period of dishonesty and devious, secretive behaviour. It took a while for me to be trusted to be left alone when I ate, especially as during recovery I'd have wobbles and relapses where I would revert back to my old behaviour momentarily.

Regaining trust starts with small steps and builds. As I say above, continued suspicion is unpleasant and can be detrimental for your child's mental health going forward, so regaining trust is important for all of you.

Dealing with guilt

Guilt, for all parties, is a common side-effect of an eating disorder. I felt guilty for a very long time – in fact as soon as I felt I wanted to get better, guilt started creeping in. I talk about guilt as a positive sign in Tough Cookie and in other chapters in this book, because actually that shows that the person inside is getting stronger and stronger – their personality is showing through again. Eating disorders don't feel guilty – hence the lies and the callous behaviour.

But generally guilt isn't good for anyone. My guilt consumed me ad actually contributed to the feelings and beliefs I held before I developed Anorexia about being a 'bad person', 'worthless', 'hated' etc. I think the reason for my later mental illness was the fact that these beliefs went unresolved – and were added to by my experience with Anorexia. So how can you combat guilt, for yourself and for your child?

Recognise that nobody is at fault

Although this has already been mentioned, it's worth repeating that there is absolutely nobody to blame in this. No single person is at fault – an eating disorder is an illness, and its manifestation has been hard on everyone involved. Once things are starting to get better it's futile and actually harmful to start going over what happened and why with an aim of pointing the finger.

Whenever a child is poorly, especially if there is a mental health issue, parents are in the spotlight and often feel guilty, even if no one has made them feel that way. Sometimes however you may be given a helping hand. It's very unhelpful to guess at causes and assume that parents have roles to play when in fact their actions are unrelated, because then as a parent your energy is focused on feeling bad and compensating and defending yourself rather than looking after and supporting your child.

Even if you've found yourself berated or belittled by friends, family, teachers or even medical staff remember that you are not to 'blame' for what has happened – nobody is at fault.

Let go of the past and move forward – live in the present, and concentrate on the future

Philosophers and psychological studies have shown that guilt is largely down to an individual being overly focused on the past. When you live in the past constantly, you can't enjoy the present – let alone look forward to the future. This theory can be applied to everyone in all walks of life, but it's especially poignant and relevant for families and individuals who have been through a prolonged period of stress induced by a mental or physical illness like an eating disorder.

Once you let go of the past, you may find it creeps up on you now and again. You may find that deep down, subconsciously, you believe that you could have done more, should have said this, shouldn't have done that. However the more you focus on what's happening right now in the present, the less the past will come to haunt you.

The Last Word

I always include a 'last word' section in my books as it's much easier to flick to one page for a reminder when you're feeling stressed, anxious or don't know what to do rather than re-reading the whole book. It's also unlikely that you'll keep everything you've learnt in this book in your mind at all times. Here are the three main things to remember when you're supporting your child or young person with their eating disorder:

1/ Your child and their eating disorder are separate

It will be difficult to remember this all the time – but this is very important as it enables you to support and help your child whilst combatting the eating disorder. Also remember that a little kindness goes a long way.

2/ Get as much support as you can

Make sure you keep trying to get medical and psychological support for your child, even if you are repeatedly turned away. Remember that there are charities and other organisations who may be able to help you. Call on family and friends if you can to support you.

3/ Look after yourself

It's going to be impossible for you to support your child if you aren't looking after yourself – as the stress of an experience like this can take its toll physically and mentally. Source counselling or specialist support if you need to, and try not to give yourself a hard time as this will only make things worse.

12. Resources and further reading

"We researched a lot ourselves and internet searches were how we first realised that Rose had Anorexia. After that we struggled to find advice and support – but there is so much more out there now." - Alison

Here I've compiled a range of resources which I hope you'll find useful. Although more are available, these are websites, charities and organisations I have had a positive experience with or have heard to have helped others.

Organisations and Charities

NHS

The NHS website has a range of useful, impartial articles including *What is Anorexia? What is cognitive behavioural therapy?* and *Symptoms of Bulimia*, in addition to information on the resources and pathways available.

ANAD

This is an American charity but the site does have some useful information for anyone seeking further advice and support.

Mind

Mind are a great mental health charity based here in the UK, and they do deal with eating disorders as well as a range of other mental health issues. You can find factsheets in addition to help and support for you and your family by contacting your local Mind or taking a look on their website.

SANE

Like Mind, SANE deal with a wide range of mental illnesses, but they do offer support for people with eating disorders also through their blog and forum facilities.

DocReady

This is a handy site which you may find useful when first visiting the GP, or for subsequent appointments so that you remember to talk about everything you need to. It can be easy to forget what you wanted to discuss when you're stressed and flustered, so DocReady offers free sheets to fill out so that you know what you are going to say and to remind you what you want to get out of the appointment.

Tough Cookie

Tough Cookie is the name of the blog I set up to help people with Anorexia by sharing my own experience and proving that it is possible to live a healthy, happy life after going through an eating disorder – even without conventional support. As well as the blog itself I often talk to young people and raise awareness of Anorexia in a positive way. I've also written several books as well as this one, which you can discover more about below.

Further reading

I wrote my books to help other people with a range of issues I have experienced myself over the years during and after my eating disorder. You can learn a more about them, read the blog or purchase the books at **www.toughcookieblog.co.uk** or Amazon worldwide.

Tough Cookie

Anorexia: The Bare Bones

Tough Love

Nutrition in a Nutshell

Recipes for Recovery

& Recipes for Recovery: The Sweet Stuff

Second Chances (a book about emotional resilience for young people written by Geraldine Hills in which I share my insight about mental health and coping strategies)